DISEASE OF
THE SPLEEN

DISEASE OF
THE SPLEEN

by
J. COMPTON BURNETT, M.D.

Author of
"Consumption", "Liver", Ringworm", "Gout", "Stunted
Children", "Organon Diseases of Women", "Diseases
of the Skin", "Change of Life in Women",
Enlarged Tonsils", "Tumors"

B. JAIN PUBLISHERS (P) LTD.

USA—Europe—India

DISEASES OF THE SPLEEN AND THEIR REMEDIES CLINICALLY ILLUSTRATED

9th Impression: 2019 .

Published by Kuldeep Jain for
B. JAIN PUBLISHERS (P) LTD.
B. Jain House, D-157, Sector-63,
NOIDA-201307, U.P. (INDIA)
Tel.: +91-120-4933333 • Email: info@bjain.com
Website: www.bjain.com

Printed in India by
B B Press Noida

ISBN: 978-81-319-0596-8

PREFACE.

The strength of a chain is equal to that of its *weakest* link, and similarly the value of a person's life may be equal to that of his *weakest* vital organ: here the particular organ is equal in importance to that of the entire organism.

Even where the tissue state of the entire organism is everywhere equally bad, it may be a life-saving act to relieve the particular organ that *first* gives way, so that time may be gained to alter the entire crasis or the quality of the stroma.

Death itself is often at the start in a particular organ, *i. e., local,* and if the part be saved in time life may be preserved. In the acute processes the value of a particular organ strikes one often very forcibly, there may be no need of any constitutional treatment; the one suffering part may be the whole case. And in many chronic cases certain organs claim, and must have, special attention. This is my standpoint in the following pages on DISEASES OF THE SPLEEN. As Forget says, *"Entre la nature médicatrice et la nature homicide il n'y a souvent que l'épaisseur d'une oponévrose."*

I deem it necessary to guard myself against misapprehension in one or two particulars. In the first place, I understand by organ-remedy *not* a drug that is topically applied to a suffering organ for its physical or chemical effects, but a remedy that has an elective affinity for such organ, by reason of which it will find the organ itself through the blood. For instance, an astringent applied to a mucous surface to get rid of a catarrh is no organ-remedy in my meaning, it is no example of Rademacher's organopathy.

Then I do not put forward organopathy as an idea of my own, or as something new, but as that of Hohenheim, and of his co-doctrinaires, as resuscitated, extended, elaborated, and systematized by Rademacher, in the early part of this century. Honor to whom honor is due; poor Hohenheim has been maliciously befouled and meanly robbed long enough, and it is high time he should have the credit of his own genius, as well as of his own folly.

The modern father of organopathy is Johann Gottfried Rademacher, who was born on the 4th of August, 1772, and died on the 9th of February, 1850. His great life-work bears this title: "RECHTFERTIGUNG der von den Gelehrten misskannten verstandesrechten ERFAHRUNGSHEILLEHRE der ALTEN SCHEIDEKUNSTIGEN GEHEIMAERZTE, und treue Mittheilung des Ergebnisses einer 25-jahrigen Erprobung dieser Lehre am Krankenbette, von Johann Gottfried Rademacher." The preface to the 1st edition is dated 1st April, 1841.

This is the work I so often refer to herein, and from which I translate the part on diseases of the spleen, though slightly condensed.

Further, I do not regard organopathy as something outside of homœopathy, but as being embraced by and included in it, though not identical or co-extensive with it. I would say—*Organopathy is homœopathy in the first degree.* And, finally, I would emphasize the fact, that where the homœo-pathic simillimal agent covering the totality of the symptoms, *and also the underlying pathologic process causing such symptoms,* can be found, there organopathy either has no *raison d'etre* at all, or it is of only temporary service to ease an organ in distress.

J. COMPTON BURNETT.

SOME OF THE LITERATURE RELATING TO ORGANOPATHY WHICH I HAVE CONSULTED.

---

1. "Der Bücher und Schriften des Edlen Hochgelehrten unnd Bewehrten Philosophi unnd Medici Philippi Theophrasti Bombast von Hohenheim Paracelsi genannt: jetzt auffs new auss den Originalien und Theophrasti eygener Handtschrifft so viel derselbigen zu bekommen gewesen auffs trewlichst und fleissigst an Tag gegeben; Durch Joannim Huserum Brisgoium, churfürstlichen Cölnischen Rath und Medicum." In 2 vols. Franckfort, Anno MDCIII.

2. Numerous writings of the Paracelsists—Crollius, etc.

3. Rademacher's Work.

4. "Zeitschrift für Erfahrungsheilkunst." Von Dr. A. Bernhardi und Dr. F. Loffler. 1847-48.

5. "De la généralité et de l'unité de la maladie." Par le Professeur Forget de Strasbourg. Reprint from *L'Union Médical*, December 25, 27, 29, 1855.

6. "De la Doctrine des Etats Organopathiques; de la nomenclature organopathologique." Par M. Piorry. Paris, 1855.

7. "De L'Element Spécificité en Thérapeutique." Par le Professeur Forget. Paris, 1858.

8. "De l'autonomie ou Indépendence de la Médecine. Ce qu'il faut entendre par Doctrine Holopathique." Par M. Marchal, de Calvi. Paris, 1860.

9. "Holo-iatrie et topo-iatrie. Discussion entre MM. Fleury et Marchal (de Calvi)." Paris, 1860.

10. "Discours sur Organicisme, le vitalisme et le psychisme." Par M. P. A. Piorry. Paris, 1860.

11. "Continuation de l'historie et de la critique.

11. "Continuation de l'histoire et de la critique Marchal, de Calvi. Pinel. Paris, 1861.

12. "Die direkte Kunstheilung der Pneumonieen." Von Dr. Carl Kissel. Eilenburg, 1852.

13. "Handbuch der physiologischen Arzneiwirkungslehre." Von Dr. Carl Kissel. Tübingen, 1856.

14. "Handbuch der speciellen Pathologie und Therapie." Von Dr. Carl Kissel. Erlangen, 1863.

15. "Dreissig Jahre Praxis. Erfahrungen am Krankenbett und im arztlichen Kabinet mitgetheilt von H. L. von Guttceit." 2 vols. Wein, 1873.

Diseases of the Spleen.

———

From the time of Morgagni's *De Sedibus,* etc., but more particularly with the introduction and generalization of physical and regional diagnosis by Auenbrugger, Laennec, Skoda, Piorry, and the mighty host of their disciples, practical medical men have been led to consider each organ by itself much more than ever before, and this often apart from medical doctrines. We may say the first half of this century thoroughly established the absolute essentiality of regional diagnosis. This separatist practice has gone so far that the organism has not unfrequently been lost sight of altogether.

Piorry in his *Traité de Plessimétrie et de l'Organographisme,* etc. (1827 to 1851), very justly remarks: "Le pathonomisme n'a donc été possible qu'à cause de la doctrine sur laquelle il est fondé."

With the direct diagnostic delimitations of the various organs by palpation, percussion, and auscultation came the coining of the words organopathy, organogeny, organography, and such like terms, which, we must say, are both sensible and useful, though organopathy had with and ever since Hohenheim constituted the backbone of the medical practice of certain, in their days mostly heterodox, practitioners, and some of them great masters of healing.

If it be asked, What is here meant by ORGANO-PATHY? my reply is, that organopathy is the specific local action of drugs on particular parts or organs, as first systematized by Rademacher in the early part of this century. It is thus, a very convenient term in therapeutics as well as in ætiology and pathology. In pathology the term organopathy has long been in general use, particularly on the Continent of Europe. The French understand by *Organopathie* an organ disease, and as such it is an accepted term in pathology. The same is true of *Organleiden* in the German language. All this by the way.

In this little work, therefore, the word organopathy is used as a technical term of *drug therapeutics;* it was copied in this country some years ago from Rademacher, and from the Rademacherian writers of Germany, without a single word of acknowledgment. But the real father of organopathy in essence and substance is Hohenheim, an eminent and learned physician commonly called Paracelsus, for proof of which see his works, and hereafter in this little volume on *Diseases of the Spleen,* if ,space permits. Organopathy is *included in* the wider generalization known as homœopathy; for whereas organopathy claims only that certain drugs affect certain parts curatively, preferentially, or specifically, as, for instance, *Digitalis* the heart (therapeutic organoapthy.), homœopathy claims that not only does *Digitalis, e. g.*, affect the heart specifically (therapeutic organopathy), but to be curative the natural disease of the organ (noso-logical organopathy) must be *like* in expression to the therapeutic organopathy or drug-action.

Homœopathy may be said to be based upon organopathy, for a drug to cure the heart of its disease specifically must necessarily affect the heart in *some* manner. But the homœopath specializes, and says further: The drug that is to cure the heart must affect the heart, certainly—that is one of the foundations of our whole therapeutic edifice, but that is not enough; the nosological organopathy and the therapeutic organopathy must be and are *similar*. And inasmuch as we can know disease only by its subjective and objective symptoms (its language), it follows that the two organopathies must be symptomatically alike, though possibly antipathic in their *mode* of action as against one another.

My reason for considering Diseases of the Spleen from the organopathic standpoint lies not only in the fact that I already worked on the same subject ten years ago, but because I believe, my experience in this field is somewhat unusual, and likely to be instructive to my readers; and incidentally I wish particularly to emphasize the fact that organopathy was a well-established system of medicine long years ago, and is no child of our time.

No doubt it wants precisioning and developing, and I trust this little volume will work a little in this direction; but for any man to come forward nowadays and pose as the discoverer of organopathy, in either name or substance, presupposes an amount of ignorance that makes one fairly stagger with amazement. I am not maintaining that treating an organ affection by an organ remedy after the manner of Hohenheim, Rademacher, and their respective co-doctrinaires, will stand as a medical system sufficient in itself, but that it is eminently workable, and is largely of the nature of elementary homœopathy, is, in fact, specificity of seat.

Neither am I unmindful of the part played by the *universalia* in Hohenheim medicine, or of the *genius epidemicus morborum.* I leave them here largely out of consideration, on the principle of doing one thing at a time.

Finally, I am very far from supposing that in the vast majority of cases an organ disease exists primarily and permanently by itself independently of the organism; on the contrary, I know well from close observation of nature that the part and the whole are commonly qualitatively the same. The organ which, to my mind, is the most systemic is the skin; and, on the other hand, the spleen has clearly a very distinct life of its own, and its own sufferings may be, and are well pronounced.

Whether any particular value is to be attached to the doctrine lately proclaimed by certain clear-seeing people that the spleen is the storehouse of vital energy I am unable to say; but I am much struck with the teaching of Rademacher, that a very large percentage of dropsies are curable by spleen remedies.

I beg no one of my readers will confound what I here say with *local treatment* of disease. I am thinking and writing about self-elective specific treatment, not local treatment.

The whole organism may suffer, or a part of it, and when such part or organ is wrong in its life and being, it generally speaks and lets its owner know, and that in its own way. The altered state of the organ sometimes produces a sense of tightness, or fulness, or pain in its own immediate vicinity; at other times, it expresses itself vicariously through another neighboring or distant organ. First come first served is a good maxim, and is generally acted upon also in diagnostics. If a man coughs, his lungs are wrong; if he gets palpitation, his heart is at fault, always to the extent of being the seat of the symptom, though not necessarily its primary one, for the symptom COUGH, PALPITATION, may arise

2

from the prompting of another organ or part either near or distant. In other words, an organ may speak out complainingly, either because it is wrong itself—*organopathically*; or it may be moved to express itself on behalf, or at the instigation of another organ —*synorganopathically;* or of the entire organism— *holopathically.*

Thus I desire to approach 'the subject of *Diseases of the Spleen* from the standpoint of *organopathy.*

From the earliest childhood of healing it has always been more or less known that, *e. g.,* to cure a liver disease you will want a liver medicine, the organ suffering being the *organopathy.*

But, as I have already said, we must ascribe to Hohenheim the honor of a real practical organopathy;* that is to say, that certain internal organs of the body seem at times to be afflicted by themselves primarily, as it were, on their own account *organopathically,* whereby the very existence of the organism itself may be threatened, other organs or parts being, or not being, consecutively involved *synorganopathically;* and that there are in nature certain remedies that have a more or less pronounced elective affinity for these self-same organs or parts which, indeed, have long borne the name of *organ remedies.* But of this more further on. To Rade-

---

* See Rademacher.

macher himself, as we have just seen, is due the formulation and actual clinical demonstration of this organopathy, for which see his work published some sixty odd years ago. Rademacher began to investigate organopathy in the year 1815, and practiced organopathically with immense success for about thirty years and to the end of his life.

Rademacher had a number of disciples who followed him in practicing, developing and defending organopathy. These disciples formed a school, and are known in literature as Rademacherians—at least that is what I call them—for it were almost more in accordance with fact to say that literature has misunderstood or ignored them, though here and there a literary freebooter has "discovered" from their store house. For a time these disciples of Rademacher held together, and published a journal, entitled *Zeitschrift für Erfahrungsheilkunst*, which began in 1847 at Eilenburg, being edited by Drs. A. Bernhardi and L. Löffler, and carrying as motto— *"Medicina ars experimentalis"*—which is very old, very hackneyed, and still as true as ever! I do not know how many years it ran, but not many, for as soon as the Rademacherians began to try to gain fixity for their indications they wandered off into the field of experimental pharmacology, but found it already occupied by—whom? by the homœopaths! and as in the case of so many wanderings, the wanderers never came back, but remained in the *field of provings* side by side with the followers of Hahnemann. Of course, before Hahnemann's time no arrangement of drugs based on provings could be made.

Hohenheim's orpanopathy, as interpreted by Rademacher, differs, therefore, somewhat from the organopathy of Rademacher's followers, inasmuch as these practically gave up the idea that remedies are *per se friendly* to the organs, and brought into their organopathy the Hahnemannic proving of drugs on the healthy, and this being done, the organopaths (Rademacherians) and the homœopaths marched side by side, the former giving up their journal.

Rademacher's work has been both ignored and criticised, but it remains classic for all time; I believe his direct art-cures of disease are unsurpassed, nay, never equalled, in the written history of medicine so far as the same is known to me.

I sometimes regret that the disciples of Hahnemann and those of Rademacher became so closely assimilated, for it seems to me that drug provings are not everything, and I cannot help thinking that had the Rademacherians kept by themselves, they would have taught us much of the higher physiology of the various organs that we still have to learn. And I am bound to say that some of the organ remedies of Rademacher possess a direct healing power over organ diseases that their provings in no way explain. Perhaps further knowledge will throw light on this; we must accept the fact, and wait for the explanation.

In daily life we make certain acquaintances with our fellow-beings, and some of these pass out of sight for a time, or for ever. Months or years roll by, and we meet with some of them again, and as So-and-so is with us, we introduce our friend to him, remarking that we have known him ever since a certain memorable event. We find that with a physician diseases and drugs stand out as so many individual acquaintances along the path of his professional life; if he meet a congenial brother chip he will very soon run off the first subject of conversation and begin to "talk shop." Most people will join in a very hearty condemnation of "talking shop," but, nevertheless, the genuine man will not be long with you before you can form a pretty correct opinion of his walk in life. Let two medicoes meet for a little social chat, and you will not have to wait long for the sign of the leech. And why should it be otherwise? Do we really expect a plant-loving botanist to prefer astronomy as a subject of conversation?

Some time since I was casually sitting in a pretty garden with a gentleman. Left a few moments together we began to chat, and the gentleman asked if I could discern a bar across the attic window. No, was my reply. "I can," said he, and almost immediately he inquired whether I had been to the Academy. No, I had not. And then in a twinkling he exclaimed: "Oh, what lovely tints, just look at the shade of the plum-tree across the path, and that green, I mean there just by the nut-tree." Need I say he is an artist?

I had not noticed any of the pretty things to which he called my attention, but I *had* seen a small issue —a tiny aperture in his skin covering his larynx.

As a striking clinical acquaintance, there stands out in my professional path a remedy called *Ceano-thus Americanus,* which acquaintance has increased with years, till it and I have become fast friends, to the advantage of not a few. Through my clinical friend *Ceanothus Americanus,* I have perhaps paid much more attention to the spleen than I otherwise should, and it is of the spleen that I am about to discourse.

As an introduction to "Diseases of the Spleen," I cannot do better than reproduce a portion of what I wrote on the subject of this *Ceanothus Ameri canus* in 1879.

ON CEANOTHUS AMERICANUS IN ITS RELATIONS TO DISEASES OF THE SPLEEN.

For several years I have been in the habit of using this drug in true Rademacherian fashion as an organ remedy. The perusal of Rademacher's *Magnum Opus* is one of the greatest literary treats that ever fell to my lot; based on Hohenheimian bizarries, avowedly and obviously merely an attempt at reducing his genial erratic *pretended* mysticism to the concrete form of a practice of medicine, by depolarizing it, if I may so speak, it is nevertheless the most genial and most original production it is possible to find in medical literature. It is the most bare-boned, lawless empiricism that one can conceive, and yet there are two leading ideas running through the entire work, and these are the *genius epidemicus morborum* and organopathy; and, considered from the pharmacological side, the other two ideas of universal (general) and particular medicines. For Paracelsus there were only *three* universal remedies, and so also for Rademacher and for their followers. Hahnemann has but *three* fundamental morbid states—psora, syphilis, and sycosis. Von Grauvogl has but three constitutions of the body—they might have all been working out the fatherlandish proverb, *Aller guten Dinge sind drei!*

The *genius epidemicus morborum* is beyond question a fact in nature, but it is dreadfully eel-like, hard to get a grip of. The same may be said of Hahnemann's tripartite pathology and of Grauvogl's three constitutional states.

Rademacher's organopathy (that an otherwise able modern writer appropriates with child-like *naivete*) is no more and no less than the homœopathic specificity of seat, with just a dash of a mystic psychic something in the several organs; if we set aside this little particular soul for each organ, it is only local affinity, or elective affinity. And it is quite true in nature, and the mind that cannot, or will not, recognize it, is wanting in catholicity of perception; and *in practice will often go a mile when three paces would have reached the goal.* Whatever else *Cantharis* may be, it is first and foremost a kidney medicine; whatever else *Digitalis* may be, it is primarily a heart medicine; and let *Belladonna* be what it may, it is before all things an artery medicine, and just in this sense *Ceanothus Americanus* is a spleen medicine.

The spleen constitutes a dark corner in the human economy, whether considered physiologically or therapeutically * I have heard it professorially

---

* "Qu'est-ce que la rate? Telle est la question, assezétrange, posée depuis trois mille ans dans la science, et dont, apres trois mille ans, la science a jusqu'à ce jour, vainement attendu la solution."—*Bourgery.*

very ably argued that the spleen is the principal manufactory of our blood corpuscles. I have heard that theory equally ably and professorially refuted, and in its stead the thesis set up that the spleen is, as it were, the *ultimum refugium* of the old and effect blood corpuscles, wherein they are .broken up, and their *débris* sent off again in the circulating medium. A third argued that all this was veritable nonsense, as the spleen had nothing whatever to do with either making leucocytes or breaking up their reddened descendants, that in fact the spleen had no other function than to act as a reservoir for the blood— being, indeed, a kind of living sac in the side, to swell or shrink according as the circulation required more or less of the circulating fluid.

I fondle this latter theory myself, and like to call it mine; whose it really is I do not know Perhaps some of my readers will be able to say what they think the spleen is good for beyond serving as the anatomical something that supposedly sends our dear fellow-countrymen in shoals off London Bridge into the Thames on a rainy or foggy day—I mean, of course, *le spleen!* This great bugbear of our Gallic and Germanic brethren—as applied to ourselves *bien entendu!* for they consider it essentially a *morbus Anglicus.* just as we like to think it is principally those naughty French who commit suicide—is really only another name for being "hipped," or suffering from an attack of hypochondriasis, and there cannot be any sound reason for refusing it a habitat under the *left* ribs, since so many have welcomed it under the right ones.

My first and only literary acquaintance with *Ceanothus Americanus* is the very short empirical account of it in Hale's *New Remedies*, which I read some five or six years ago. Previously I had frequently felt a difficulty in treating a pain in the left side, having its seat, apparently, in the spleen. *Myrtus communis* has a pain in the left side, but that is high up under the clavicle; the pain that is a little lower is the property of *Sumbul;* still lower of *Acidum fluoricum;* a little further to the left of *Acidum oxalicum;* more to the right of *Aurum;* right under the left breast of *Cimicifuga rac.*

These remedies promptly do their work when these left-sided pains are a *part* of the disease-picture, but they will not touch the pain that is deep in behind the ribs of the left side; more superficially *Bryonia* has it; a little deeper than *Bryonia, Pulsatilla nuttal,* will touch it; and so will *Juglans regia,* which poor Clothar Müller proved as a student. But the real splenic stitch requires *China, Chelidonium, Berberis, Chininum sulphuricum* or *Conium,* or *Ceanothus Americanus.*

Some years since I treated a lady for "violent vomiting, pain all up the left side, cough with expectoration, profuse perspiration, and fever." She was not a native of the place, but came only for a short visit, and took lodgings in a small house facing a meadow on the banks of the river; the locality was at one time a part of the port, but was many years ago reclaimed. At my first visit she told me she often got inflammations on the chest with cough, and finding considerable fever, cough, pain in left side, and dulness on percussion of the same side, I quickly ticketed it *pleuro-pneumonia sinistra,* and gave *Acidum oxalicum,* which seemed to cover all the symptoms, and to correspond also to the supposed pathological state within. *Oxalic acid* somewhat relieved the vomiting, but nothing more, and I then gave various remedies, such as *Aconite, Bryonia, Phos., Ipec.,* and thus elasped about three weeks, but patient remained as ill as ever. Then I went into the case with very great care, and examined my patient very thoroughly, and, see, there was *inflammation of the spleen.* I gave her *Ceanothus Americanus* in a low dilution, and all the symptoms, subjective and objective, disappeared right off, and my previously ill-treated patient was sitting up in a week, and quite well in a few more days. I had never before met with splenitis in the acute form, and, indeed, it is a very rare disease in this country.

Cases of chronic pains in the spleen occurred subsequently in my practice, and they rapidly yielded to

Ceanothus, one of which I well remember; it is this:—

Chronic Splenitis.—A young lady of about 26 consulted me for a chronic swelling in the left side under the ribs, with considerable cutting pain in it. She stated that it was worse in cold damp weather, and she always felt chilly; the chilliness was so severe and long lasting that she had spent the greater part of her time during the previous winter sitting at the fireside, and now she was looking forward to the winter with perfect dread. In the summer she had felt nearly well, but the lump and the chilliness and pain nevertheless persisted, but it being warm, she did not heed it much, it being quite bearable.

Ceanothus Americanus quite cured her of all her symptoms, and subsequent observation proved its permanency. Often during the following winter she called my attention to the fact that she was not chilly and felt well.

Another case which I treated at a later date was that of a young man somewhat similarly suffering.

Chronic Splenitis.—This young man had been sent to my dispensary, and was occupied in the post-office in some light but ill-paid employment. His whole trouble consisted in *severe pain in the left side in the region of the spleen,* and he had long vainly sought relief of many, probably àt dispensaries. He therefore put in an early appearance at my new dispensary to try the new doctor, probably on the well known principle of the new broom. He had become quite low-spirited and began to fear he would become totally unfit for work, and naturally that was a very serious matter for a young married man. He told me he had formerly helped his wife in her household matters, doing the heavy rough work, but the pain in his side had now become so bad that he could not carry a bucket of water into the house or even sweep up their little yard, as handling the broom pained him so dreadfully. I was pressed for time, and prescribed *Ceanothus Americanus* in pilules of a low dilution, and promised to go into his case that day week, meaning to percuss the part and ascertain whether the spleen was enlarged. He returned that day week almost well, and the following week was quite well. At my request he again reported himself some time afterwards, and he still continued well.

I resolved to *begin* my next case with a physical examination. My next case was this—

Chronic Hypertrophy of the Spleen.—A middle-aged lady consulted me, shortly after the above case, for a *severe pain in the left side and a large swelling in the same position.* Remembering the last case, I said I must examine the side. She objected, so I declined to treat her; then she said she would think about it and consult with her husband on the subject. In a fortnight or so she returned (driven by the severe pain in the side), and I examined the side and found an enormous spleen occupying the entire left hypochondrium and reaching inferiorly to about an inch above the crest of the ilium; it bulged towards the median line and ran off to an angle laterally. It was of long standing.

Gave *Ceanothus Americanus* in a low dilution.

This lady being very intelligent I begged she would allow me to examine the side again after I had finished the treatment. She promised to comply.

Fourteen days after this she came full of gratitude, and reported that the swelling was smaller and the pain considerably less.

To continue the medicine. She never consulted me again, but as she was a near neighbour of mine I often saw her, and somewhat six months afterwards she called to pay my fee, and then informed me that she had soon got rid of the pain entirely and the swelling was much smaller, so she had discontinued the medicine altogether, and did not deem it needful to trouble me again.

This is the usual thing. People will not be at the trouble of seeing the doctor as soon as they are better, they seem not to understand any interest one feels in the case. We can only make periodical reliable examinations of patients in a hospital; in private practice it is extremely difficult, as all practitioners know to their chagrin. Still, *faute de mieux*, we must put up with these fragments. This patient has had no children, and had a very fresh complexion.

My next case is also one of *Chronic Hypertrophy of the Spleen,* though only about half the size of the one just narrated. Subject: a poor woman of about 30 or 32 years of age, whom I was requested to see by a very kind-hearted benevolent lay minister. She is the mother of several children, very poor, ill-fed, and over-worked, but withal a good, respectable woman, and very clean. She had a considerable and very painful swelling in the left side under the ribs, that had been there for some time, and latterly she could not get up on account of the severe pain. I carefully examined the tumor and satisfied myself that it was a very much swelled spleen, and the pain seemed to me to be due to its pressing against the ribs. I marked its size on the skin with ink, made her engage not to wash off the ink mark, and promised her I would call in a week, having first prescribed *Ceanothus* as in the other cases. But the fates were against my laudable plan, for I received a message, the day before my next visit was due, to the effect that Mrs. ———— felt herself so much better that she was up at her housework, and begged me not to call again, as she thought it unnecessary.

Since then I have at times had cases of deepseated pain in the left side to treat, and have mostly found it yield to *Ceanothus,* though not always. In one case in which it failed the pain was cured with *Berberis vulgaris.*

In one case of jaundice, characterized by very severe pain in the *left* side, I gave *Ceanothus,* with very prompt relief of the pain only; *Myrica cerifera* then finished the icterus. Before giving the *Ceanothus* I had given *Chelidonium majus.*

In one case of severe metrorrhagia characterized by pain in the left hypochondrium, *Ceanothus* gave instant relief to the pain, and checked the hæmorrhage. It failed me in a subsequent similar attack in the same person, when *Conium* was effective.

Chronic Splenitis, Chills, and Leucorrhœa.— Some four years since, perhaps a little more, I treated a lady of about 55. She complained of rigors at frequent intervals, and pain in left side, both of long standing.

The leucorrhœa had lasted some twenty years, and was profuse, thick, and yellow. She had been for years under the best allopathic physicians of her native city, and finally given up as beyond the reach of medical art, evidently on Molière's principle that "Nul n'aura de l'esprit ques nous et nos amis."

Nevertheless, the patient bethought her of Homœopathy, and came under my care. Her last physician had finally suspected cerebro-spinal mischief, and hinted at incipient paralysis.

The pain in the side was the most prominent and distressing symptom, and for this I prescribed *Ceanothus*. In a month the pain was entirely cured, *and also the leucorrhœa,* while the cold feeling was very much diminished, but not quite cured. I have also never succeeded in quite curing it with any subsequent treatment. I watched the case for nearly four years, and am thus enabled to state that the pain in the side and the leucorrhœa never returned, and the chilliness never again became very bad, but still she had it a little when I saw her last.

CASES OF ENLARGED SPLEEN MISTAKEN FOR HEART DISEASE.

A few years ago I was attending some of the members of a family of position in London, and at my various visits I occasionally heard of an invalid daughter of the family suffering from a hopelessly incurable disease of the heart, for which she was said to be under a West-End physician, who was thought to devote himself especially to diseases of the heart. The heart was said to be enormously enlarged, and the patient had had to give up first dancing and then hurrying, and finally she was only allowed to walk very slowly and carefully, lest the

3

hugely enlarged heart should rupture. Several physicians had examined the case, and all were agreed as to its cardiac nature. I had never seen the young lady, and took no particular interest in the frequent narrations of her heart troubles; they are common enough. Time went by, and the mother used to speak of her "poor invalid daughter" with increasing despondency, finishing up one day with the remark that the unfortunate girl was no longer allowed even to walk, as the doctor considered even that now fraught with danger.. "Is it not sad?" said she. "Would you like to see her?" I declined, saying, I never cared about seeing other physicians' patients.

More time elasped, and finally I was requested to take the case in hand. I demurred at first, because such hopeless cases are as unsatisfactory as they are painful.

At last I consented to take over the case, and I appointed a time to call and examine the patient.

During all my professional life, I have rarely been more taken aback than I was after I had made my examination of the patient, for I found the heart not only not enlarged, but of the two rather abnormally *small*, although apparently the cardiac dullness extended a foot down the left side. But this dulness on percussion was due to an *enlarged spleen* which pushed up the diaphragm and left lung by its bulk, till the heart and the spleen gave one continuous dull percussion note. Patient had many genuine symptoms of real heart disease—dyspnœa, palpitations, inability to lie on the left side, faintness—but these were due to the mechanical hindrance to the heart's action produced by the spleen bulking upward so much.

That young lady I met three weeks ago looking blooming, and as agile as possible, and she has done her share of dancing, tennis, etc., for some years.

Ceanothus Americanus cured the enlargement of the spleen for the most part, though it swelled again two or three times at some months' intervals, and *Ferrum phosph., Conium, Thuja, Berberis,* and other splenics, came into play before patient was really well. Looking at the case now with the advantage of wider experience and more matured views of biopathology, and with the patient fully six years under my observation, I regard the affection as a primary disease of the leucocytes due to vaccinial infection, the spleen being disturbed secondarily, and then the heart mechanically. I am confirmed in this view by the fact that the spleen would not leave off swelling up at certain times till I had cured the vaccinosis. That prince of splenics, *Ceanothus Americanus,* readily cured the splenic engorgement, but did not touch the blood disease which caused it. This is the inherent defect of organopathy, that it is not sufficiently radical in its inceptive action, but the like remark applies to every other pathy more or less, because the primordial cause is more or less elusive, and generally quite beyond positive science, which only admits of what it knows, and will not seek to encompass the unknown by the processes of thinking and reasoning. Because in former times philosophy made science impossible, the votaries of science now round upon philosophy, and sneer it out of view. To trace back proximate effects to remote causes is now ridiculed in medicine because *mere* science is productive of gross-mindedness, incapable of following the *fine* threads of the higher perception.

It was also about the same time that I was at the house of a patient in London, the wife of a general officer and the conversation fell upon the general's heart affection, and also upon that of their *char-woman*. I learned that the lady of the house took a certain interest in her charwoman because she had seen better days and had an invalid husband depending on her labor more or less. This charwoman was, it was said, suffering from an incurable disease of the heart, causing her terrible distress; on rising in the morning she would have to fight for her breath, so that it would take her often three-quarters of an hour to get dressed, having to pause and rest from the dyspnœa and its effects, nevertheless she persisted in thus getting up and dressing, and did as much charing as she could get. Her pride would not allow her to beg of her friends. Such was the story, and I really felt curious to see the charwoman, and promised to do what I could, though from the account given me by the general's wife, I certainly thought it quite a hopeless case.

Calling a few days later, I saw the lady and the charwoman, and having duly examined the latter, I promised to cure her! She was to come to my city rooms, and report herself every fortnight. On returning from the bedroom to the drawing room, the general's wife accused me of cruelty in thus raising the poor old woman's hopes "when," exclaimed she, "you *must* know it is impossible." I tried to explain that it was a case of enlarged spleen, and not the heart disease at all, that the charwoman was suffering from, and that the palpitations and fightings for breath were the mechanical sequels of the splenic engorgement, but my patient evidently did not believe it, for she wound up by saying, "As you will treat her for nothing, I hope you may succeed, and it is very kind of you, but you must know that the poor woman has been under various doctors, and all have declared it incurable heart disease, and I merely wanted you to tell me of something to relieve and ease the poor old thing."

This was towards the middle of October. A

careful physical examination showed that ' the heart-sounds were normal, but there was much beating visible in the neck, and the heart's action was labored. In the left hypochondrium there was a mass corresponding to the position of the spleen, and a dul percussion note was elicited not only in the left hypochondrium, but also in the right, and all across the epigastrium, or pit of the stomach, from side to side.

The following notes were put down at the time: "Heart-sounds, normal; apex beat, exaggerated; splenetic dulness extending up to the left mamma; the whole region very tender, so much so that she cannot bear her clothes or any other pressure." The prescription was: *Ceanothus Americanus* 1x ℥ij, five drops in water three times a day.

November 14.—Has been taking the *Ceanothus* five weeks to-day, and has taken altogether three bottles of it, viz., ℥vj. It has nearly stopped the pain in the left side, *which had lasted for quite twenty-five years.* This pain came on suddenly, especially if she drank anything cold. She would get an indescribable pain under the left ribs, and she would have to fight for breath, and the dyspnœa would be so severe that it could be heard in the next room, frightening everybody. She had ague thirty years ago in Northamptonshire Repeat.

November 29.—Not much pain left; the cold feeling still there, but nothing as it was. Repeat.

December 20.—Has the pain in the left side, but very little; *has not had any of those attacks of fighting for breath;* she can walk better, and the side is much smaller, which she knows from her dress. In her own opinion she is less in the waist by two inches. Before taking the medicine, for very many years she was compelled to pause in the morning when dressing, and lie down on account of the beating of the heart, but this has all gone; on examining by palpation and percussion I find the dulness diminished by four inches in the perpendicular, and by about the same from side to side. However, there is still some tenderness on pressure, and the swelled spleen can still be felt towards the mesian line and inferiorly. She can now do her work (charing) very much better. ℞. *Tr. Ceanoth-Am.* 1, four drops in water three times a day.

January 10.—The pain is gone; has now no pain in walking, and she is a great deal stronger and better. The coldness in the pit of the stomach has gone. Repeat.

February 7.—In the left hypochondrium there is now nothing abnormal; the old ague-cake has disappeared, there being no dull percussion note. Her own conception of the size of that portion of the enlarged spleen that used to stretch across the pit of the stomach to the liver is thus expressed by her: "I used to say it was as big as a half-quartern loaf."

Not only is the lump gone, but she is much stronger; she now wears stays again, and fastens her clothes with comfort. She again gets some cold feeling in the pit of the stomach, but not much. Her liver seems considerably enlarged, and there is still too much beating of the blood-vessels (veins) in the neck. In my opinion the condition of the blood-vessels calls for *Ferrum* 6, which I now prescribe, and when that has done its duty—as it surely will— the liver will call for attention. But what I wanted to bring out was the specific affinity of *Ceanothus Americanus* for the spleen, and its consequent brilliant effects, as the *simile* only grounded on the homœopathic specificity of seat, which some say has no existence.

This poor woman thus took *Ceanothus* during about four months in small appreciable doses: at first the 1x and then the 1 centesimal.

The existence of the hypertrophy was ascertained by percussion and palpation; and subsequently I ascertained by the same means that it had ceased to exist. Although patient took the drug for four months I could not find that it affected any other organ—liver, kidney, bowel—save and except the spleen.

The dyspnœa and palpitation were cured certainly, but these arose, I submit, from the engorged condition of the spleen itself.

As far as I could ascertain, the secretions and excretions were not affected in the least degree; the remedial action must, therefore, be considered specific. My conception of the cure is simply this, that the specific *Ceanothus* stimulus persistently applied restored the spleen tissue to the normal. This homœopathic specificity of seat suffices only in simple local disturbances; it is only a *simile,* not a *simillimum.* The latter would, I apprehend, have affected the liver also and the right heart, and I should then not have needed further detail treatment.

This charwoman continued to attend at my rooms for some months, and *Ceanothus Americanus* and other indicated remedies cured her of her "incurable heart disease;" and I saw no more of her for some time, when one day she was ushered into my consulting room. She came up to where I was sitting, told me she was perfectly well, could do any work with ease, and—then occurred one of the sweetest things in my whole professional life—the old lady (and *what a lady!*) put a tiny packet on my desk, tried to say something, burst into tears, and rushed out!

I never saw her again, and have often since wished I had kept that particular sovereign and had it set in diamonds.

Supposed Consumption: Chronically Enlarged Spleen.

· The case I am about to relate is not without practical interest. The subject is a fine young Anglo-Indian of about 21 or 22 years of age, who a couple of years since, commenced preparing for the study of medicine in London. His father was my patient, and told me, as he left for the East, that one of his boys, whom I had casually seen, was going to remain in London to study medicine as a profession, rather than as a hobby, as said father has done for many years.

Two years elapsed, and then my patient returned from the East, and came to see me on his own account, and I incidentally inquired about the medical student. "Ah! he is better now, but he had to give up the study of medicine, as the professor said he was going into consumption. He had spitting of blood, and they sent him to America. He has returned, and is better; but I am still anxious about him, as his breath is very short. He looks very well."

The young man came in due course, and a very careful percussion and auscultation of the chest revealed nothing but a *very* large spleen filling up the left hypochondrium, and clearly impeding both lungs and heart in their action.

I ordered *Ceanothus Am.* 1 in five drop doses.

He took the drops for a month or so, and came again on the 16th of February, 1887, telling me he breathed easily and comfortably, and demonstrated to me that he was inches smaller round the body, by showing me his waistcoat and trousers that were previously tight, but now uncomfortably loose, so much so that he laughed at their bagging. Evidently his pulmonary symptoms had never been phthisical at all, but were merely mechanical from the engorgement of the spleen.

SPLENALGIA.

A lady came to me complaining of the following series of symptoms: . . . Pain in the left side corresponding to the region of the spleen, so bad that she cannot lie on the left side; with this pain in the side there are two other disturbances, indicating that a kind of vascular turgescence—an *orgasmus humorum* —underlies the whole, viz., palpitation of the heart and piles. With these also some indigestion, and a feeling as if the visceral contents of the abdomen were being pulled down.

℞. *Ceanothi Americani* 3x ℥iv. Three drops in water three times a day.

She came from the country, so I did not see her again, but as I asked for a report in a fortnight, her husband wrote at the end of that period to say that she was well and needed no further attention.

The case of this lady rather interested me, as some six years previously she came under my care for chronic headaches that seemed climacteric; I treated her for these headaches, but could not make any impression upon them, and then, on going over the various organs, I found that the urine contained a small quantity of albumen. This our ordinary remedies removed in about two months, and the headaches disappeared. About a year later the albuminuria again returned in a very slight degree, and with it some cephalalgia; both yielded at once to the same remedies, and she had remained well till she came with the splenalgia and hæmorrhoids. I suspect, therefore, that the old albuminuria was not due to any kidney mischief, but to venous congestion of the kidneys.

PAINFUL ENGORGEMENT OF SPLEEN WITH VARICOSIS.

Some cases of varicosis will not get well till you cure the spleen of its—perhaps slight—enlargement. Thus, a hale gentleman of 70 odd consulted me early in 1887 for varicose veins, particularly below the knees. The veins on the surface of all four extremities get knotty and painful. There is a pain under the left ribs, which is worse when he has urinary urging. The splenalgia he has had these ten years.

I prescribed *Ceanothus* 1. It cured the splenalgia

and painful vein-knots in a few weeks. He is now comfortable under left ribs for the first time for ten years. He is also not so short of breath. The stricture of the urethra, of which he also suffers, was not affected by the *Ceanothus,* and he remains under my care to see if the stricture will also yield to treatment.

CHRONIC ENLARGEMENT OF SPLEEN WITH HEART SYMPTOMS.

An unmarried lady of 49 came to me in January, 1887, for a supposed affection of the heart. Being rather stout, she was thought to have a fatty heart. She complained of numbness and heaviness down the left arm for a considerable time, also of a pain under her left ribs at times ever since her childhood, and over which part she had had blisters and poultices from most of her many physicians, generally with relief for the time being. An examination showed the heart to be normal, but disclosed an enlargement of the spleen. Patient has suffered from whites all her life.

She took *Ceanothus Americanus* 1, nve drops in water night and morning, for two months: I had ordered it for one month only, but she found herself so much better from the medicine that she got a second bottle of it on her own account, and continued taking it for just two months, when she came to inform me that she felt quite well, and percussion showed that the spleen had returned to its normal size. The leucorrhœa was a trifle better, but not much, and for this affection she remained under treatment. The spleen engorgement had been cured by the spleen remedy, but the constitutional state had remained unaltered; but with this I am here not concerned.

VOMITING—CHRONIC AND SEVERE HYPERTROPHY OF SPLEEN.

On June 16, 1881, an unmarried lady of 23 years of age, residing on high ground in London, came to me saying she suffered from chronic and severe vomiting, debility and emaciation. The vomiting began about midsummer, 1880, at first once or twice a week, and it has been gradually getting worse, so that she now vomits generally about half an hour after every meal, though occasionally she will miss a meal and not vomit. She has lost 13 lbs. in weight since January last. Menses are getting scant. There is a very considerable area of dulness on percussion in the left hypochondrium, and when she is sick she feels pain under the left ribs. She often gets caught with a pain under left ribs; and besides this left hypochondriac pain, she gets a clawing pain in the pit of the stomach, not seemingly connected with it, and apt to last the whole of the day. Lifting her arms seems to pull her stomach, and hurt in the middle. Cannot wear stays, because their pressure hurts; she dons them, but is compelled to put them off every few hours. There is a clear space of about an inch between the area of dulness on percussion of liver and spleen respectively. She flushes at times. She is generally chilly, sitting by the fire when others do not, and she goes to sit by the kitchen fire when there is no fire anywhere else in the house. Cannot walk upstairs other than very slowly, because of dyspnœa. The vomit is sometimes nearly black, as if she had been drinking coffee; at times it is watery, at others just the food.

℞. *Ceanothus Americanus* 1, ʒv. Five drops in water three times a day.

She took no other remedy, and was discharged cured in about seven weeks. The patient had previously been under an able homœopathic practitioner, who had treated the case purely symptomatically, and thus failed, for the very sufficient reason that the symptoms which he treated were secondary to the engorgement of the spleen, and so his remedies all failed. God forbid that I should say one disparaging word about symptomatic treatment as such, for we but too often have only the subjective symptoms to go by, but where an exhaustive physical diagnosis is possible, it should always be made, and should stand in importance far before merely subjective symptoms, as these may be, and often are, consequently in this sense delusive.

For, in this case, it must be manifest that vomiting due to an enlarged spleen can never be cured by rémedies that physiologically produce vomiting, but by such as will bring a large spleen back to the normal.

ENLARGEMENT OF SPLEEN—AGUE-CAKE.

In November, 1886, a *poitrinaire* lady of 29 came under my observation complaining of indigestion, flatulence, and palpitation, with cough and considerable debility. The flatulence is worse in the evening. The right lung gives a dull percussion note almost all over the front aspect. There is an endocardial bruit, best heard at mid-sternum. The spleen fills the entire left hypochondrium, while in the right side the hepatic dulness runs up, seemingly almost to the nipple. There is slight increase of vocal resonance on the right side of thorax. The skin across the epigastrium is very brown. Had a cough ever since she had fever in Malta three years ago; also frontal neuralgia.

Chelidonium 1 cured the swelling of the liver, and reduced the spleen a trifle. *Ceanothus Americanus* 1 restored the spleen to the normal, but did not touch the neuralgia. *Thuja occidentalis* 30 cured the neuralgia, and I am now endeavoring to go deeper into the case to find out the etiologic x of her constitution, which causes me to state that she is *poitrinaire*, the anatomic basis of which is a sodden, phlegmy, bronchial lining; but *what* is the etiologic moment thereof?

This case also illustrates both the insufficiency of the organopathic conception and also its practical utility.

QUASI-HEART DISEASE.

A city gentleman between 30 and 40 came to see me on November 25, 1885, for heart disease, from which he had suffered for fifteen years. He has been under quite a number of eminent physicinas, tried changes to spas, and been for climatic benefits east, west, north, and south, at all times and seasons. Cruising about in a yacht does him most good. For the past several years he has been under Sir ——— for his heart.

I find his heart rather small, its action irregular an endocardial bruit most audible below and to the left of the left mammilla. He gets very chilly, and his fingers often go dead in the early morning: the so-called "poor circulation" so frequently accused. He is languid, anæmic, seemingly barely able to rise in the morning. Has been vaccinated three times, but only took very slightly the first time.

The lungs are flat; the spleen notably enlarged.

The most distressing symptom is his nocturnal palpitation.

R. *Ceanothus Am.* 1. Five drops in water three times a day.

4

After taking the *Ceanothus* thus for a fortnight, the cardiac and splenic dulness no longer ran into one another, and the palpitation and numbness were much better.

Regarding the case causally as partly from vaccinosis, I gave *Thuja* 30 infrequently, which did him so much good that he stayed away for a month. *But a very ugly patch of eczema had come out in the right axilla! and he subsequently got shingles on left thigh.*

The quasi-heart disease was gone, and has not returned, and the further course of the case presents no relevancy to my present thesis. Strange to say, the endocardial bruit had also quite disappeared.

The foregoing entirely chips from my own workshop, I think it would be well to give an example of what Rademacher's organopathy really is, by reproducing in rough and ready translation the bulk of his chapter on Diseases of the Spleen from his great life-work, the *Rechtfertigung*, already referred to.

RADEMACHER'S EXPERIENCE OF DISEASES OF THE SPLEEN, BASED ON HOHENHEIM'S ORGAN-OPATHY.*

Spleen Medicines.

It is difficult to find good spleen remedies, because the spleen, as compared with the liver is seldom painfully affected in its substance. When it pains, the pain is most commonly at the margin of the epigastric and left hypochondriac region rather than in the hypochondrium itself. But, alas! just at this very spot liver affections also often express themsleves, so this symptom is uncertain. The comfortable lying on the left side, and the impossibility of lying without distress on the right side, certainly speaks for a spleen affection, provided always that the left lung be not affected. So it is very well to pay attention to this symptom, but it is an uncertain one. People whose spleen is much affected like to lie on their backs, just as do those who have the right lobe of the liver much enlarged, and neither can lie comfortably on their sides. When we further bear in mind that the spleen (so far as we know at present) is neither an excretory nor a secretory

---

*Abbreviated from—RECHTFERTIGUNG der von den Gelehrten misskannten, VERSTANDESRECHTEN ERFAHRUNGSHEIL-LEHRE der alten scheidekünstigen, Geheimaerzte, etc., von *Johann Gottfried Rademacher.* Erster Band. 4th Edition. Berlin, 1851.

organ, it follows that we cannot. have any symptoms indicating a disturbance of such-like functions.
When we further consider that the gall ducts are
sometimes sympathetically affected in spleen com-
plaints, with the urine discolored as in gall affections—that, in fact, the *menstrua digestionis* in general are qualitatively altered; and that to fiill the
cup of difficulties to overfilling, abdominal plethora
will simulate painful spleen disease; it is easy to
see that the finding of good spleen medicines is, indeed, a very difficult affair.

The states and symptoms that, during my medical
career, I have known to arise more or less frequently
from spleen affections are the following:

Pain in the stomach (often).

Cough, and that oft, violent, and suffocative.

Bellyache (at times).

Chronic diarrhœa, and rather more frequently.

Constipation.

Asthma (seldom)

Disturbed renal functions and their consequent
dropsy.

And with regard to such dropsies, in so far as
they are not due to organismic affections, I ascribe,
according to a rough calculation, about one-third to
the spleen.

In women the spleen affects the womb and the
vagina, causing emansion, or excess of the flow,

and leucorrhœa. [This I (Burnett) have myself observed very frequently, and also a very distinct sympathy between the male urethra and the spleen, which Rademacher does not appear to have noticed, since probably peccant urethrorrhœæ were not very common in a place like Goch.]

Not a few acute fevers of a secondary nature (Consensueller Art-synorganismie) and agues are the mere concomitants of spleen disease. When abdominal affections are prevalent, we at times meet with splenic fever. But in this one year differs from another. At one time, when liver affections were prevailing, I have not had to treat a single case of spleen fever in a whole year, and at other times, liver affections still prevailing, I have had here and there an intercurrent case or two of spleen fever.

Brain affections, such as mania and melancholia, eye diseases, such as diplopia, amblyopia, chronic inflammations, I have seen arise from the liver, but thus far not from the spleen. If I had ever witnessed an epidemic of spleen affections, I should know more about the organ. As it is, what I have to say about spleen medicines can only be imperfect.

CARBO VEGETABILIS.

Rademacher speaks of the difficulty of really diagnosing a primary spleen disorder, and then says:

Continuous asthma, worse at night, is not a common complaint. It may be, like the cough, of a synorganic (*consensueller*) nature, and depending upon a spleen affection. Not long since I witnessed an instructive case of the kind. A man who, in his youth, had had a moist eruption all over his body, which eruption was fruitlessly treated with medicines, but went away of itself in adult life, but left behind an ugly fish-skin-like epidermis, began to complain of tension in the left hypochondrium, becoming at times a little painful. He did not, however, consult me for this, but for shortness of breath. I soon ascertained that he had had the tension in the hypochondrium much longer than the asthma, and so thought he was suffering from a disease of the spleen, and which I thought the more likely, as he had never had the least the matter with his lungs. Well, I did not gave this man *Carbo*, but another remedy, and the complaint got visibly better. When it had reached a certain stage of improvement, he was hard hit by a then prevailing liver fever, which in his case implicated the chest. This chest affection, however, did not consits in the previous asthmatic attacks, but in pain in the side, with cough and bloody expectoration. He got well, but hardly was he able to be up all day when the old asthma came back worse than ever. Thinking the liver complaint might not be quite cured, I gave him a good hepatic, but the asthma remained. Here

I gave him the spleen remedy—the spenic—which had done him so much good before the accute affection came on. The man asked for it himself, but it did no good at all. Asthma and cough remained, and instead of picking up after his acute disease with good nights' rest, the asthma drove him every night out of bed. I now gave him *Carbo,* which soon altered the face of things. Cough and asthma lessened; the latter soon disappeared altogether, so that the man was able to make the hour and a half walk home to his friends, who had given him up.

But not every case of asthma, due to the spleen, will yield to *Carbo.* Those stomach pains that, as they pass off, lose themselves in the left hypochondrium, and which I put down to the spleen, I have at times cured with *Carbo;* more frequently, however, with other spleen remedies.

Kidney affections, with dropsy, due to primary spleen disease, I have never tried to cure with *Carbo,* because I thus far have managed to cure them with other remedie, and I do not hold it to be right to try experiments from mere curiosity .

SCILLA MARITIMA.

In my youth I used *Scilla,* like so many other physicians, as a pectoral and diuretic. But finding it thus used so little helpful, I gave it up in contempt. During the last twenty years, in which I have taken more interest in the affections of single organs, I came to recognize the necessity of finding out good and reliable remedies proper to the various organs, and as I had indeed such a very poor stock of spleen medicines, I read one day in an old Galenic author (I really don't remember now in which) that *Scilla* was a very good splenic. Dioscorides also reckons it to the spleen medicines, but he has put down so many drugs as organ remedies that one's whole life would not suffice to try half of them. All things considered, I thought the the old Galenic's idea not a bad one, and from that time on I have used *Scilla* as a spleen remedy, and I have never given it up since.

Although I may be in some doubt as to whether *Carbo veg.* really acts healingly upon a diseased spleen, I am, on the contrary, very sure about *Scilla.* I have found it quickly and surely helpful in such painful spleen diseases—affections painful and beyond any doubt in and of the spleen.

In those dull pains on the border of the left hypochondriac and epigastric regions, there being no signs of any liver affection (a rather uncertain and negative), I have used *Scilla* as a remedy with advantage.

I have also used *Scilla* with very striking results in those so-called stomach pains that are made so much better by lying on the left side, and which in all probability depend upon a primary affection of the spleen.

Finally, I have used it with good results in one case of continuous asthma from a spleen affection, with nocturnal exacerbation, and in which *Carbo* has been used in vain, but in this case the spleen engorgement was of such long standing that I hardly believe in its being radically cured.

As too the dropsy that depends upon a diseased spleen, I no doubt gave it in former years in such also, for I dare say I gave squills to nearly all my dropsical patients; and that may account for my having found it so useful in dropsy, but I am not so very sure. But since I have had the habit of trying to find out in all diseases the primarily affected organ (provided the to-be-cured disease be not a primary one of the whole economy) I have not used it, for the very sufficient reason that I have not needed it, but of which more anon.

The preparation I prefer is the tincture 15 to 30 drops five times a day. In cases where it caused diarrhœa in these doses, I have had to come down to 5 drops three times a day.

Aqua vel Tinct. Glandium Quercus.

I became acquainted with this remedy in a wonderful way. Many years ago (I do not remember the exact time) a working carpenter, who had previously lived in Credfeld, came to seek my advice for his bellyache, which was of long standing. According to his own statement, he had long been under Sanitary Councillor Schneider in Credfeld, who was not able to help him, and so sent him to Professor Günther in Duisberg. Ten journeys thither were likewise in vain.

I tried my usual remedies for seemingly such cases, but to no good; and as I noticed he was a good cabinetmaker, and dabbled a bit in upholstery, I told him it would be a good plan if he were to hire himself out to a country squire as joiner, thinking that the food of the servants' hall would suit his sick stomach better than the beans, black bread, and potatoes of the master carpenter. The good fellow followed my advice, and lived with a squire for many years; and I heard nothing more about him. Finally, he married the parlor maid, and settled here in this town as a joiner. One day when visiting his sick wife I remembered the old story of his bellyache, and wanted to know how it then was. "All right," said he, "I have not had it for years." It seems that a local surgeon, being one day at the squire's, told him to get some acorns, and scrape them with a knife, and then put the scrapings into brandy, and leave them to draw for a day, and then to drink a small glass of this spirit several times a day. He did as he was advised, and was forthwith relieved, and very soon entirely freed from his old trouble.

From what I knew of the surgeon, I was very sure he could not give me any intelligent reason for his prescription. I should only have heard that acorn scrapings in brandy were good for the bellyache, or, at the most, I may have ascertained from what doctor, or peasant, or old wife he had got the tip.

But this would have done me but poor service; and as I had in the meantime become much more cunning, I questioned the joiner himself afresh as to the kind of his old pain, particularly as to the part of the belly where the pain was *last felt* when he had had a bad attack. He was in no doubt about it, but at once pointed to the part of the belly nearest the left hypochondrium. So I very shrewdly suspected that the abdominal pains were really owing to a primary affection of the spleen, in which notion I was strengthened by remembering that the best pain-killing hepatic and enteric remedies had done him no good.

To get as soon as possible to the bottom of the thing, I set about preparing a tincture of acorns, and gave a teaspoonful five times a day in water to an old brandy drunkard, who was sick unto death, and of whom I knew that he had suffered from the spleen for a very long time, the spleen being from time to time painful. He had likewise ascites, and his legs were dropsical as far as the knees. It occurred to me that if the acorn tincture were to act curatively on the spleen the consensual kidney affection and its dependent dropsy would mend. I soon saw that I had reckoned rightly. The urinary secretion was at once augmented, but the patient complained that each time after taking the medicine he felt a constriction of the chest. I ascribed this to the astringent matter of the acorns, and thinking the really curative principle thereof would most likely be volatile, I caused the tincture to be distilled. This acorn spirit caused no further constriction, and the urinary secretion was still more markedly increased, the tension in the præcordia became less and less, and this hopelessly incurable drunkard got quite well, much to the surprise of all who knew him, and, honestly speaking, much to my own surprise also.

Having thus put the spirit of acorns to such a severe test, and that in a case that I already knew so well, in which it was impossible to make a mistake as to the primary affection, I went further, and used it by degrees in all sorts of spleen affections, and that not only in painful ones, but in painless ones, in the evident ones, and in those of a more problematical kind. Gradually I became convinced that it is a remedy, the place of which no other can take. More particularly is it of great, nay, of inestimable value in spleen-dropsy. Later on, I found that the volatile curative principle of acorns may be still better extracted with water with the addition of alcohol. [The *aqua glandium* is thus prepared:—One pound of peeled and crushed acorns to the pound of destillate.] Perhaps water alone might extract the healing principle, but it would thus not keep, and so the cures would be uncertain, not to mention the fact that such-like decaying medicines are a great trouble to the chemists. The dose of the spirituous acorn-water (the only preparation I have used of late years) is half a table-spoonful in water four times a day. It has not much taste; some would even say it has none, but the doubter may make a solution of alcohol and water in the same proportions, and he will soon find that it has quite a taste of its own.

I must make mention of two of its peculiar effects. Certain few people feel, as soon as they have taken it, a peculiar sensation in the head, lasting hardly a minute or two, which they say is like being drunk.

With a few people, particularly with those who have suffered from old spleen engorgements, diarrhœa sets in after using it for two or three weeks that makes them feel better. It seldom lasts more than a day, and it is not weakening, but moderate. Hence it is not needful either to stop the acorn-water, or to lessen the dose.

I could add many instructive cases of spleen dropsies and other spleen affections, in which the volatile principle of acorns proved curative, but as I have so much more to say on other subjects, I dare not be too discursive on this one point; besides, what I have already said will suffice for common-sense physicians. Still I cannot forbear noticing a few bagatelles. For instance, I have found that the acute spleen fevers that occur intercurrently with epidemic liver fevers, are best cured with *aqua glandium*—at least that is my experience.

Furthermore, I am of opinion that the three splenics of which I have made mention are curative of three different morbid states of the spleen, and I know well from my own experience that acorns are indicated in the most common spleen affections; and, finally, I am not acquainted with any positive signs whereby those three separate morbid states of spleen can with certainty be differentiated from one another.

There are other spleen remedies to which I must allow a curative action in diseases of the spleen, but I have not used them so often as those, because the morbid states of which they have been more particularly curative have not occurred so often to me.

Those I have tried are—*Galiopsis grandiflora*, a celebrated spleen remedy of the old time, and not to be despised; and *Rubia tinctoria*, which is also undoubtedly justly credited with being a splenic, but I have not used it often enough myself to be able to say anything satisfactory about it.

BACCÆ JUNIPERI.

These berries are a good spleen medicine which I have often ordered for the poor, and sometimes with good effect. The berries must be crushed, and a handful left a long time to draw in four cupfuls of boiling water if you want to see any effect from them. I do not think it is the æthereal oil, but a non-volatile principle of the berries, that acts as a splenic.

OLEUM SUCCINI NON RECTIFICATUM.

This is a good spleen remedy. It must be given in small doses, and as people often make a mess of the dropping, it is best to give it in some other fluid. I order it in acorn-water and formerly in acorn-spirit. To six ounces of acorn-water I add half a scruple or a whole scruple of the oil. They do not mix chemically, but if the mixture be well shaken our object is attained; the patient does not get more into his stomach than we intend. The giving them together contains no virtue; at least I have no reason to think so. The *Oleum Succini* does good service in painful spleen affections wherewith there are convulsive attacks, such as the hysterical and hypochondriacal often have. Only once did I observe its smell cause hysterical convulsions in a woman, but that is a very rare exception to the rule.

Oswald Crollius lays great stress on the importance of rectifying the oil of amber, but what he says therein is not true. The rectified oil is nothing like so serviceable as the unrectified. In general Crollius is the most honorable ,and the most straightforward of all the jatro-chemists, but a man of but small understanding.

CONIUM MACULATUM.

The late Professor Günther, of Duisberg, used to give for chronic cough a powder composed of one grain of *Conium* and ten grains or a scruple of aok mistletoe. He had once cured an old gentleman with it. A colleague of mine, an out-and-out sceptic, who had in vain patched away at the old gentleman, did not deny the cure, but ascribed it to chance, to the particular faith the patient had in Günther, and not to the action of the powder. But I could in no wise agree with his opinion, for although I had at the time but very little experience of *Conium*, still I knew Günther was a sensible physician, who wrote simple prescriptions, and so must have understood the curative action of his medicines. I once met Günther over a patient, about whom there was little to say, as he was evidently dying. In the course of our conversation, I begged him to tell me what he thought about *Conium.* He was willing, but, being interrupted by the anxious friends of the patient, only gathered that

he set great store by it. I had several times easily
cured patients of his of liver coughs, and to whom
he had in vain given *Conium,* as I saw from the
prescriptions of his that they brought with them;
from which I concluded that it was not a sure liver
remedy. I had before fruitlessly used *Conium* in
painful spleen affections, and hence too hastily concluded, because I was still stupid, that it was not a
spleen remedy. Now that I had become wiser, and
understood that nature could produce different sorts
of spleen affections, I began also to see that while
Conium might be quite useless in one kind of spleen
affections, it might nevertheless be remarkably
curative in another kind of spleen disease. Thus I
once used it in a case of consensual cough arising
from a primary spleen disease. This is hard to
cure; all the lung medicines do no good. Of the
belley medicines, the only one that would occasionally
be of any service was the *Semina cardui.* I now
put *Conium* to a very severe test, that is to say, I
gave it in cases in which the *Cardui Mariæ semina*
failed me, and lo and behold I saw the most
beautiful and most astonishing curative action from
it. Since then I have never given it up, and as I
make no unreasonable demands upon it, it has never
disappointed me. I stated earlier on that Günther
gave it in combination with oak mistletoe, but there
is nothing in that; I have found it just as active with

5

sugar of milk or sweetwood, as when triturated with oak mistletoe.

MAGNESIA TARTARICA.

My readers will not much care to learn how I became acquainted with this remedy. So I may just say that I neither stole it from a brother brush, nor did one very kindly communicate it to me, neither did I find it in a book. Still it is manifestly a remedy with which a spleen affection may be ousted. I confess, however, that I knew nothing of it till four years ago, and, from want of opportunity, have not used it much. But as I have got rid of painful spleen disease with its aid, and that such as would not obey other remedies, I am bound to conclude that there must be a spleen affection in nature which is peculiarly subject to the healing power of this remedy. It does not follow that because this particular disease has come comparatively seldom under my observation that this will necessarily be the case in the future.

I have not yet given this remedy in those spleen diseases that are evidenced by consecutive cough or dropsy, for the very good reason that other and twice better known remedies sufficed. I never try experiments with new remedies until the old ones leave me in the lurch.

The average dose of the remedy is one scruple four or five times a day. In this dose it has no laxative action. Should one, however, meet with very sensitive bowels, whose movements are increased by this dose, less must be given, for I have observed that the laxative action does not hasten the healing.

Rademacher also favorably mentions *Cicuta* and *Acidum pyroligneosum* as topic splenics.

There is not much to be learned in any English works that I have read on spleen medicines. I, personally, know nothing of—

LUFFA ECHINATA.

Moore (*Diseases of India*, 2nd edition, p. 527) narrates that Dr. Dickinson (Bengal Service) had some years ago recommended the *Bindaäl Rerula*, or *Luffa echinata*, an indigenous plant of the N. O. *Cucurbitaceæ*, as a remedy in spleen disease, and says that he himself had used it in dispensary practice with apparently good results.

I may now refer to a little of my own clinical experience with Rademacher's spleen remedies, and particularly as to the *Oleum Succinatum non rectificatum*, which has rendered me brilliant service, as my readers will see.

CHRONIC ENLARGEMENT OF THE SPLEEN WITH HEMIHYPERÆSTHESIA, CEPHALALGIA, DYSPNŒA, ORTHOPNŒA, CONVULSIONS.

A more remarkable case of its kind I never observed. Subject: A young lady towards the end of her teens, of good family, and at a finishing school

In London. Had been treated at home for hysteria of a severe type both homœopathically and hydropathically, the latter consisting of the cold douche when a convulsive attack was on. The cold douche was only once applied, and nearly killed the patient. Many months after it was applied, when the patient was in a state of what seemed to be approaching death from exhaustion with violent delirium, she literally yelled at what she imagined was some one approaching the bed to throw water on her. It would fill a little book to give a complete history of her case; so I will summarize it as briefly as may be.

At first, and for a year or two, I treated her for *attacks*. Said "attacks" I had never seen, but I put them down as a form of epileptoid seizure, though it was distinctly stated that the convulsions were mostly left-sided. Sometimes violent palpitation of the heart was essentially the attack; at other times dyspnœa, orthopnœa; and always a pain in the left side under the ribs, going up and down: and patient, no matter how violent the convulsive attacks, was never quite unconscious. I was not able to see an attack, and could never get a really clear description of them. "Dreadful fighting for breath" coming on in attacks, with pain in the left side, was the essence of all the descriptions given to me. I treated the case, but without doing any real good, and finally she was seized with an attack so violent that the parents telegraphed from the country to me to know what to do, and I felt it too serious a case to be treated by me at a distance, and so I wired back that I resigned the case to their family physician, himself an eminent homœopathic practitioner, who also had formerly tried his hand at the case, but in vain.

Many months elapsed, and I heard only indirectly about the case; and then the friends, in sheer despair and disgust at the obstinacy of the attacks of what their family physician said was a severe form of hysteria that would not go away for good, but ever and anon came like a domestic explosion, creating unrest and tension, brought her to reside near me in the neighborhood of London, and this was at the beginning of the winter of 1886-'87. The attacks soon came, and I had the opportunity of observing them. On entering the room I thought I heard steam coming out in short, sharp "whists" from a kettle-spout, but I found it was patient's expiratory efforts. The dyspnœa was very great, and the convulsions most violent, being always confined to one side—the left—but varying as to position on the trunk, being at times in the nape, then on a level with the nipple, then in the lumbar region, sometimes so bad that the body would be bent like a hoop, and the movements very often sent patient flying either against the bedstead, over on to the next bed, or on to the floor; and hence we had to pad all hard objects. Some of the convulsive contortions were awful to behold, and most of her friends devoutly hoped and prayed that she might die. For some weeks I was the only one who believed recovery possible, so long, so violent, and so exhausting were the convulsive attacks. Myself, I only lost heart once, and that was after a series of attacks of convulsions lasting for hours, and leaving only short intervals. Her friends several times fetched me, in the night, believing patient to be dying.

The thing went on for months, and I was able to get slowly at some constant characteristics.

1. When out of the attacks patient was comparatively well in herself, and looked well, only as time went on, and the attacks lasted for hours with great violence (relays of two, and sometimes three persons being required to hold her down), she became very weak from exhaustion.

2. The appetite was poor, the tongue coated, the bowels obstinately confined.

3. The left side of the body (trunk) was so tender that she could not bear the least pressure. Touching it gently with one finger even made her wince.

4. The spleen was considerably enlarged, and the whole region excessively tender.

5. She had a *constant* fixed pain in the left half of skull, worst about midway between ear and the sagittal suture, and she usually held her head in left palm.

6 Warmth was agreeable, and cold aggravated very distinctly, and particularly frost and snow; violent attacks always came on whenever it froze. "Thunder has always tried me."

7. There was pronounced periodicity, sometimes irregular, but also at times and for weeks together as regular as a clock, there being two, three, or four attacks in twenty-four hours.

I could not agree that the case was one of hysteria, as the family physician thought. In the very early part of the treatment I treated her for epilepsy, but did her no good. Then, in view of the enlarged spleen, I gave *Ceanothus Am.* and other spleen remedies but in vain.

She was at times feverish, and had *Aconitum;* very flushed in the face, and I ordered at first *Belladonna,* and then *Lachesis,* but in vain.

Phosphorus, Gelsemium, Zincum, Cuprum, Ignatia, Nux, Puls., and many such were equally useless. *Aranea diadema, Cicuta,* were no better.

Sulphur and *Plumbum* did a little temporary good, and we thought *Cuprum* and *Acid hydrocyanic.* eased the convulsions a little, and, also *Mikania guaco.* Essentially they did no real good.

The fixed, constant, and often severe pain in the
left side of the head at last compelled me to assume
the presence of a tumor in the brain, perhaps of a
vascular nature. *Silicea* and a number of other
remedies were given on this hypothesis, but the patient
seemed practically uninfluenced by them.

Heretofore I had treated the case from the particular
standpoint, as well as from that of the entire
organism, and had failed, so I thought over the case
afresh, and came to the conclusion that Rademacher's
account of the action of *Oleum Succini* made
that drug appear a likely remedy. I threrefore
prescribed the non-rectified oil in five-drop doses
three times a day. That was early in March.
. . . In forty-eight hours the convulsive attacks
ceased, and in three weeks the hemihyperæsthesia.
The pain in the head—in fact, the whole series of
morbid phenomena—slowly disappeared. So I am
now disposed to regard the case as a primary disease
of the spleen from the very beginning, the
convulsions and head pain being consecutive thereto.
This is the *kind of cure* one meets with in Rademacher,
and which gave the tone to his life and
practice.

When I say *kind of cure,* I mean an obviously
bad case of disease not mending of itself, and cured
straight off—generally jugulated. Evidently, too,
Hohenheim used his organ remedies, so that he

effected striking cures; any wonder that he became overbearing and arrogant?

After taking the *Oleum Suc.* tor six weeks I very carefully percussed and palpated the left hypochondrium, which was no longer tender, and the enlargement of the spleen had quite disappeared, though patient said the side was *at times* tender still, and the pain in the head still persisted a very little. No convulsion since the second day of taking the *Ol. Succini.*

LEUCOCYTHÆMIA SPLENICA.

There is nothing quite certain about this diseaseform, except that scholastic medicine defends it as a distinct morbid species, and then- -declares it to be incurable.

A consideration of it in brief will not be out of place in a treatise on *Diseases of the Spleen.* That there are cases answering to the ordinary description of splenic leucocythæmia is quite certain; several such cases have come under my observation, two of which are now under my care and are getting better— incurability notwithstanding.

Splenic leucocythæmia has been defined as hypertrophy of the spleen, with an alteration of the blood consisting in a considerable augmentation of the number of the white corpuscles. Virchow called this disease *Leukamie* (from ευκα, μιολαν, white, blood), because of the alteration in the blood. Now that the white blood corpuscles are often called leucocytes (λευκος , white, κυτος , cells), Bennett's name of leucocythæmia (splenica) is likely to carry the day as against Virchow's leukamie, though, perhaps, not in Germany.

The disease is variously called a cachexia, a diathesis. The first case recorded is that of Dr. Craigie (1841), and then Hughes Bennett and Virchow run neck and neck in their claims for priority; and, I think, to Bennett belongs the honor. The year 1845 may be accepted as the year of the recognition of the new disease; and for years medical literature gave it a front place, but of late one sees but a very occasional note on the subject. Whether leucocythæmia splenica is essentially different from other varieties of leucocytosis remains to be investigated; and whether common anæmia and it are degrees of the same is also very much an open question. Perhaps future progress in our knowledge of hæmatology may show us as very numerous, diseases, the one *anæmia*, that "calls for iron" For I apprehended that if the spleen be the breeding place of some of the leucocytes, and the lymphatic glands and the bone-marrow the breeding places of other leucocytes, we shall necessarily have three varieties of anæmia, namely, the splenic, the lymphatic, and the medullary— causally, perhaps very different.

Then the spleen is said to be the place where some of the red blood corpuscles are broken up and destroyed. If this be true, then there must in all probability be two distinct forms of lecocythæmia splenica—the one due to formative lack, and the other due to undue splenic destructiveness. The probability of the truth of this speculative theory is greatly enhanced by the absolute uselessness of the ferric medication in some cases of anæmia; whereas in others the striking, nay, almost startling, curative results following the same treatment surely characterize it as different.

Clearly, the anæmia which yields to iron must be very different from that which does *not* yield to it.

I have found *Oleum Sussini non restificatum, Spiritus glandium Quercus, Thuja* 30, *Mangan. acet.* 1, and *Natrum sul.* of positively curative effect in leucocythæmia splenica.

Beyond any question there is a form of leucocytosis that is surely and rapidly cured by iron, a remedy which the Paracelsists considered *universal, i. e.,* affecting that which is common to the whole economy (the microcosm), and not having any particular affinity for any one of the organs of the body above another. It follows, therefore, that from Hohenheim's standpoint iron would be no remedy for leucocythæmia splenica unless the disease was one of the entire organism (or its blood), and, indeed, iron is no remedy in leucocythæmia splenica; and I regard the therapeutic uselessness of iron in a bad form of anæmia as a first step to the diagnostic differentiation of the *kind* of leucocytosis one is dealing with. Nevertheless, good authorities claim that iron will reduce the spleen, but this may be by reason of its unquestioned action on the blood.

I have found it of considerable therapeutic advantage to regard leucocythæmia as being causally connected (often remotely) with vaccinosis and gonorrhœa—to me a great clinical fact, but on which I have here nothing further to say. And, indeed, *cui bono?* The world that would not listen to Autenrieth Hahnemann, Grauvogi, Wolff, H. Goullon, and others, would also not listen to me.

Well, we can wait; and since the spleen, on which I have been here already too discursive, is the *organon risus* of the ancients, I must keep my own functionally intact, and hence will close with their old distich—

Cor sentit, pulmo loquitur, fel continet iras,
Splen ridere facit, cogit amare jecur.

PART II.

A medical man practising in the Fen District came to see me a year or so ago, to consult in regard to his own health, and before departing he desired to thank me for my little book about *Diseases of the Spleen.* Said he, I have increased my practice very considerably since using *Ceanothus,* as I find it readily cures the spleen cases, which abound in my neighborhood. I cannot, he continued, make use of your little doses, for many of my patients would simply laugh me in the face. So I use an infusion in ordinary doses and cure splendidly.

In order to ascertain whether larger doses than those I had been in the habit of using would cure without causing any inconvenience, I have given latterly in spleen affections five or ten drop doses of the mother tincture of *Ceanothus* several times a day, and, with a very few exceptions, I find it acts curatively just as well as the smaller doses, and causes no inconvenience. However, in a few cases, I had to go back to my former smaller doses, as the larger ones caused pain in the left side and sometimes palpitation. This is entirely in accordance with all my experience in the use of organ-remedy, viz., wherever the degree of homœopathicity is at all pronounced, the dose must be small. In ordinary cases where there is only specificity of seat, *i. e.,* homœopathicity of the lowest degree, small material doses are the best and the most rapidly curative. The medical man just referred to, promised to give me his experience of *Ceanothus.* Here is what he kindly sent me:—

"Anything fresh to-day?" I asked, as I sauntered into No. 12 Warwick Lane.

"Yes!" said the genial secretary, handing me *Diseases of the Spleen,* by Compton Burnett.

"I promptly bought the volume, as I knew absolutely nothing about the therapeutics of this *terra incognita* to the ordinary and extraordinary, orthodox, allopathic, semi-allopathic, and semi-homœopathic practitioner. It was the best investment I ever made as, all unknown to myself, the Fen District of Cambridgeshire, in which I resided, was full of spleens (abnormal). After perusing the work I realized my appalling ignorance.

"Let me give one or two cases:—

"Visiting a resident patient one day twelve months ago, I got into conversation with a lady visitor living in Newmarket, who informed me that the previous ten years of her life had been spent mostly in bed or on a couch. Heart disease, her family physician had diagnosed, as well as several professors. I informed her after having made a rapid physiognomical diagnosis that she had a very good heart, and that she could be cured in probably a few months.—Tableau

"After four month's treatment she was nearly well and stopped treatment for three months. An attack of Influenza brought on the old spleen trouble again, but six weeks' treatment brought her round again. There was slight ovarian complication in this case.

"I used *Ceanothus Americanus* with a small dose of *Chel.*, and she liked it flavored with *Am. carb.* and *Tinct. capsici.*

"I have usually two spleen cases every week—sometimes more Sometimes the spleen is very much enlarged and always painful—sometimes complicated with tender left lobe of liver, and also the latter enlarged, and *Ceanothus* has in every instance hitherto removed the spleen trouble, and I have only failed in one case of enlarged and tender left lobe of liver, associated with enlarged and painful spleen. *Ceanothus* has cured the latter, but as yet, this liver baffles me. I put it down to my own ignorance."

Turning over the leaves of the *Homœopathic Recorder* of May 15, 1900, I saw something about my old friend *Ceanothus,* and which I forthwith proceed to commandeer.

CEANOTHUS.

(BY J. C. FAHNESTOCK, A. M., M. D,)

"I wish to call the attention of the readers of the *Medical Century* to a very valuable remec y; a remedy very little used by most physicians and possibly never by many—*Ceanothus.*

"This oversight is not strange, as it has only been used empirically, and no proving has ever been made of it so far as I know. Its principal and almost sole use has been in splenitis, where it has accomplished much good.

"During last summer and this winter I made several provings of *Ceanothus.* To my surprise the first symptoms noticed was a sticking pain in the spleen, and after the continued use of the remedy, there was quite an enlargement of that organ, worse by motion, but at the same time unable to lie on the left side; following this there was pain in the liver, a congestion and enlargement, with sticking pains worse by motion or touch.

"Pain in lumbar region, with a desire to urinate.

"The prover for several days and nights was unable to get any rest, owing to these aggravating pains in the sides; when lying on left side the pain in the spleen was so great I could not lie still, and upon turning over I experienced the same difficulty on opposite side. At this time the urine had a green color, bile being found in the urine, urine frothy, traces of sugar with an alkaline reaction, sp. gr. 1030.

"Pain and weak sensation in umbilical region. A generally weak sensation. Pain and soreness in muscles on exterior part of thighs noticed in every prover.

"Tongue coated in the centre with a dirty white coating. Loss of appetite. Loss of flesh was noted in one prover, with general weakness, and paleness of face.

"Stools become clay-colored, showing an action on the liver.

"One prover who had malaria several years ago developed a beautiful case after a somewhat prolonged use of the drug.

"Every physician using *Ceanothus* in splenitis following malarial fever knows full well its wonderful action. Where the spleen is affected from any cause, with enlargement, deep sticking pains, worse by motion, but at the same time unable to lie on left side, the case will generally yield quickly to *Ceanothus.*

"I have at the present time a case of pernicious anæmia, accompanied by spleen pains, rapidly improving from the use of *Ceanothus.*

"I would suggest the remedy in question for leukæmia, pseudo-leukæmia, splenic anæmia, and Hodgkin's disease. Also, for the so-called bilious attacks, the patient having a dirty white coating on tongue, pain in liver and spleen, with or without clay-colored stools, possibly with pains in umbilical region, and with it all a general tired feeling.

6

"When this drug becomes thoroughly known it no doubt will be a great remedy for malaria and its effects."—*Medical Century*.

RUBIA TINCTORIA IN SPLENIC ANÆMIA.

Splenic anæmia is often hard to cure, so, indeed, is any case of anæmia which will not readily yield to the action of iron in some form. The truth is anæmia is very often effect, and the cause is hard to get at.

A couple of years ago I was called upon to treat a case of splenic anæmia after influenza in a young married lady. It would yield to nothing; eminent physicians tried their hands after the family doctor had in vain done his best. I tried, but also in vain. The late Dr. Swan, of New York, once wrote me that he had found *Med.* (high) a good antidote to the ill effect of influenza, which statement I have very frequnetly verified. It failed here. When we were all in despair (residence at the seaside had also failed) I bethought me of the fact that pigs fed on modder get their tissues colored red, and on that idea I gave Mrs. X. 60 drops of *Rubia Tinctoria* θ in water daily. She picked up immediately, the extreme pallor yielded, the dyspnœa lessened, patient and her husband were loud in their praise of the remedy and begged to be allowed to continue it, which was done, and a perfect recovery was the result.

In several such cases of anæmia I have used the *Rubia Tinctoria* with great advantage. As I have before stated, *Rubia Tinctoria* was one of Rademacher's splenics. I call to mind the case of a maiden lady of 52 years of age, who was brought to me in February 16, 1899, for anæmia and debility of a very obscure nature. There had been no period for six months. I prescribed *Rubia Tinctoria* θ, 10 drops in water night and morning. In six weeks she declared herself nearly well. The medicine was continued, and in another two months she was discharged cured.

CEANOTHUS IN CONSENTANEOUS HEART DISEASE.

Where the heart is perturbed consentaneously with a spleen affection, the relief obtained from the use of *Ceanothus* (and other splenics) is often very noteworthy.

The number of cases of spleen affections commonly reported as cardiac is very considerable. And even in cases where the heart is really at fault, the easing of the spleen region by splenics is often a great help to the comfort of the heart.

Thus a patient of mine who suffers from valvular disease these many years consulted me anew, in the spring of 1900. The valvular condition was, of course, unalterable, and the heart distress was pretty bad from supercompensatory hypertrophy; the greatest distress was under the left ribs, and patient was often chilly, and, moreover, in his youth he had had ague.

A few drops of *Ceanothus* two or three times a day brought very great relief, so much so that patient became very loud in its praise, and continued taking it for three months. He told me yesterday that no medicine he had ever taken had ever brought so much comfort to his heart: "The palpitation has almost ceased, I can lie down flat in bed, and can sleep lying on either side, and I pass much more water." Where the congestive distress lies in the liver region, hepatics play a similar part, as this gentleman's remark to me proved, when he said, "I remember you used to give me *Chelidonium*, but that was when the pain used to be in the right side, and that is why I always keep some *Chelidonium* by me in case."

Testimony as to the therapeutic value of *Ceanothus* is coming in from many parts; the following case from Dr. R. T. Cooper, of Wimpole Street, is of very great value:—

"DEAR DR. BURNETT.—The influence of *Ceanothus Americanus* upon enlargements of the spleen receives such interesting confirmation from the following case, that I am sure it will gratify you.

"A cabman, aged 50, living at Boscombe, near Bournemouth, who had been operated on some two years back at the Brompton Cancer Hospital for what appears to have been enlarged spleen, wrote to me in the beginning of August under the following circumstances:—

"It sems that this man and Marrell, whose case of cancer of the pylorus I refer to in my work on *Cancer and Cancer Symptoms,* had occupied adjoining beds in the hospital, and he, having met with Marrell, whose case had been looked upon in the hospital as quite hopeless, immediately started for London to consult me.

"As he arrived too late, he subsequently wrote me a letter which I received when on my holiday, and which I answered on the 13th August by forwarding a prescription of *Ceanothus Americanus* θ gtt. vii; aq. ʒij, five drops four times a day in water.

"From his letter, as well as from an interview with him on 12th September, I gathered these particulars.

"He had been dragged forward by a bolting horse when driving, and the bar of the phaeton had pressed heavily upon the diaphragmatic region, and this was followed by severe pain, especially in the splenic region, which swelled up and became more and more painful. After suffering in this way for a year, he was admitted to the Cancer Hospital, and after being there for a month, was operated on for enlarged spleen. Before the operation the pain was very great, and certainly the operation relieved this, but after the operation he continued to get weaker and weaker, and his weight went down; in the two years since then he has lost two stone, and is becoming more and more enfeebled. His face is florid, and blood rushes to his face and head, making the face scarlet and the eyes blood-shot and dim, and he staggers with weakness. He has to hold on to things when standing, and then the lower part of his body and legs gets cold and his hands and fingers numb. A vein running up the right temple enlarges, especially in the morning, to the size of his little finger. The local sensations are thus described in his letter:—

" 'Now as to the place where the operation was, it seems to bubble up, relief coming from pressure, and if it do not work like this, I am worse. Then under my ribs the left side is like a bird fluttering.'

"On 12th September he came up from Boscombe to see me, having taken two bottles of medicine. His testimony then was that he was better in every possible way, and that whereas, before taking the medicine, he could not do the lightest yard work for three hours together, he could now keep at work all day. The vein on the right temple had not shown up since he began the *Ceanothus,* and the urine, which before had been thick and scanty, was now clear and free. The bowels were acting naturally, though sleep was poor. On examining the side I found a dull hard mass posteriorly and immediately below diaphragm, and a hard band 2 in. by 2 in. in front, just above the extensive scar of the operation and below the diaphragm.

"The inference from local examination would be either that the entire spleen had not been removed, or that new growth had taken place since the operation. Anyway, the distinct and pronounced relief given by the *Ceanothus* could not be questioned.

"I may mention there was no history of anguish seizures or of chills and perspirations at any time of the disease."

URTICA URENS AS AN AGUE MEDICINE.

The stinging nettle is a splenic of very high order, as I have elsewhere proved. I will content myself with giving one case of ague cured by it.

CASE OF AGUE CURED BY URTICA URENS.

A young officer, 29 years of age, was invalided home from Burma with malarial fever and a swelled spleen in the spring of 1893. He had had quinine, arsenic, and iron, but was not improving or free of fever.

March 2.—℞. *Urtica urens* θ; ten drops in water night and morning.

March 16.—No fever at all; much sediment in urine (quite normal).

May 20.—No fever.

June 22.—No fever. Discharged cured.

As I have entered so largely into the question of the value of *Uritica urens* in my booklet, entitled *Gout and its Cure,* I will refer my readers for further information hereanent to its pages.

DR. CLARKE'S CEANOTHUS CASE.

One Sunday morning about a year ago an American lady brought her daughter, aged 14, to me, complaining of a severe pain in the left side. They had just arrived in London, having landed at Liverpool a day or two before, and the history of the case was this: During the voyage, as the patient lay in her berth, she stretched over to reach something in the cabin, and was immediately seized with a violent stitching pain in the left side. It was thought at the time that the pain would soon go away, but it did not. And after landing, the pain persisted and grew rather worse, so that the plans of the family, which were to proceed to the Continent in a few days, were jeopardized.

As it is always well to localize exactly a pain or an ailment whenever possible, I asked the patient to undress, and I found that the pain was not in the chest wall or abdominal muscles, as the history would rather suggest it to be, but was deep in—in the spleen, in fact. Moreover, percussion showed that the spleen was quite considerably enlarged. The pain was $>$ by lying on the painful side.

As it was Sunday and the pharmacies were likely to be closed, I put a powder of *Ceanothus* 30 on the patient's tongue there and then, and gave her a prescription for the same medicine to be made up later on, with instructions to come and report on the Tuesday following. She came in due course, and reported that in two hours from receiving the dose the pain had gone—before the prescription was made up. I again examined the side, and the splenic dulness had gone back to normal.

So we see that my original claim for *Ceanothus Am.,* that it is a homœopathic remedy in the ordinary sense is substantiated.

INDEX

Acidum fluoricum, 14.
    ,,   oxalicum, 14.
Ague-cake, case of, 36.
Ague cured by urtica urens, 75.
Anæmia, splenic, cured by rubia tinctoria, 70.
Aque vel Tinct. Glandium quercus in diseases of the
                          spleen, 45.
  ,, ,,   ,,   ,,   ,, how prepared, 46.
Aurum, 14.

Baccæ juniperi a good spleen medicine, 51.
Belladonna is an artery medicine, 12.
Brain affections sometimes arise from the liver, 41.
Bryonia, 14.
Burnett's Dr. Compton, experience of Rademacher's
    spleen remedies, 60.

Cantharis is a kidney medicine, 12.
Carbo vegetabilis in diseases of the spleen, 41.
Ceanothus Americanus, a medical man's satisfactory
                      experience of, in the Fen
                      district of Cambridgeshire,
                      65.
    ,,   ,,   Dr. Clarke's case of, 76.
    ,,   ,,   notice regarding, in *Medical
                      Century*, 57.
Chelidonium in enlargement of spleen, 36.

Chills, case of, in lady of, 55, 20.

Clarke's, Dr., ceanothus case, 76.

Conium maculatum as a remedy in spleen disease, 52.

Consumption, supposed, case of, 30.

Cooper, Dr. R. T., on the therapeutic value of ceano-
    thus Americanus, 72.

Crollius, Oswald, on rectifying the oil of amber, 51.

Digitalis is a heart medicine, 12.

Ferrum in disorder of the blood-vessels, 28.

Galiopsis grandiflora in disease of the spleen, 50.

Hale's new remedies, 14.

Heart disease, quasi, case of, 37.

    ,,   ,,   ,, consentaneous relieved by ceano-
            thus, 71.

Homœopathy is based upon organopathy, 3.

Hohenheim the father of organopathy, 4.

      ,,   his organopathy differs from Rade-
            macher's, 8.

      ,,   his organopathy the basis of Rademacher's
            experience, 39.

Iron, a curative in leucocytosis, 62.

Juglans regia, 14.

Leucocythæmia splenica, consideration of, 61.

Leucorrhœa, case of, in lady, 55, 20.

Literature relating to organopathy, viii.
Luffa echinata, a remedy in spleen disease, 55.

Magnesia tartarica, a remedy in spleen disease, 54.
Mangan. acet. 1 in leucocythæmia splenica, 62.
Medical Century on ceanothus Americanus, 57.
Moore, on luffa echinata, 55.
Myrtus communis, 14.

Natrum sul. in leucocythæmia splenica, 63.

Oleum succini non rectification a good spleen remedy,
      51, 55, 60.
Organopathy, literature relating to, vii.
      „   what is meant by, 2.
      „   technical term of *drug therapeutics,* 4.

Piorry, his remarks in *Traité de Plessimêtrie,* etc., 1.
Pulsatilla Nuttall, 14.

Rademacher, his teaching on dropsies, vii.
      „   his disciples on organopathy, 12.
      „   his organ remedies, 8.
      „   his experience of diseases of the spleen,
                based on Hohenheim's Organopathy,
                39.
      „   Dr. Burnett's experience of Rademacher's
                spleen remedies, 60.
Rubia tinctoria in splenic anæmia, 70.
      „   „   a splenic, 71.
      „   „   case of maiden lady of 52 cured by, 71.

Scilla maritima in diseases of the spleen, 43.

Semina cardui as a belly medicine, 53.

Spiritus glandium quercus in leucocythæmia splenica, 63.

Spleen, case of chronic hypertrophy of, in middle-aged lady, 17.

,, ,, ,, ,, ,, ,, in poor woman, 19.

,, ,, ,, inflammation of the, 15.

,, case of chronic enlargement of, with hemi-hyperæsthesia, cephalalgia, dyspnœa, orthopnœa, and convulsions, 55.

,, chronically enlarged, supposed consumption, case of, 30.

,, chronic enlargement of, with heart symptoms, case of, 33.

,, enlarged cases of, mistaken for heart disease, 21.

,, enlargement of, ague-cake, case of, 36.

,, medicines, 39.

,, painful engorgement of, with varicosis, cases of, 32.

Splenalgia, case of, 31.

Splenitic stitch, medicines required for, 14.

Splenitis, chronic cases of young lady, 16.

,, ,, ,, ,, young man, 16.

,, ,, chills, and leucorrhœa, in lady 55 years old, 20.

Sumbul, 14.

Swan, Dr., of New York, on influenza, 70.

Thuja occidentalis in neuralgia, 36.
   ,,   30 in leucocythæmia splenica, 63.

Urtica urens as an ague medicine, 75.

Vomiting, violent, with pain on left side, case of, 14.
   ,,   chronic and severe hypertrophy of spleen,
        case of, 34.